The 5-2 Diet Guide to Weight Loss

Easy 5-2 Diet Recipes and Secrets to Lose Fat

Table of Contents

Introduction

I want to thank you and congratulate you for downloading the book, *"The 5-2 Diet Guide to Weight Loss – Easy 5-2 Diet Recipes and Secrets to Lose Fat"*.

This book contains proven steps and strategies on how to successfully lose weight with the 5-2 Diet. You will learn many amazing, easy to make recipes that are aligned with the 5-2 Diet and will help improve your energy and lose weight.

Thanks again for downloading this book, I hope you enjoy it!

How the 5-2 Diet Works

The 5-2 diet requires dieters to limit their consumption of calories for two non-consecutive days a week while eating regularly on the remaining days. It is said to be beneficial in weight loss and promoting overall health.

General Tips for Dieters

With this diet, men are allowed to consume six hundred kilocalories while women are allowed to consume five hundred kilocalories during fasting days. Food portions should be controlled while on this diet in order to achieve the maximum effect.

Of course, you should also learn how to plan your meals accordingly. Meal planning is essential while dieting. It lets you know how much calories you are eating, as well as enable you to make good food choices.

You should never mistake the typical fasting with 5-2 fasting. In general, people do not eat or drink anything when they fast. With the 5-2 diet however, you will only limit your food intake during your days of fasting.

If you make not eating during your fasting days a habit, you will be at risk of developing health issues, not to mention that you will also be more prone to weight gain. Not eating actually reduces your metabolism, so by not eating properly, more fats will be stored by your body.

In addition, you should realize that spreading out your calorie consumption throughout the day is the best thing to do. This will keep you from getting hungry on different times of the day.

Eating several times a day is more advisable than eating three times a day. When you eat three full meals, you can and will get hungry until your next meal and will be forced to snack. If you eat five to six small meals a day, you will prevent hunger pangs and other unnecessary cravings.

During your non-fasting days, you can eat anything you want. There is practically no limit on what you want to have for breakfast, lunch, dinner, and snacks. Of course, if you want to achieve weight loss faster, you should still make healthier food choices.

As much as possible, avoid eating processed foods. Refrain from eating fast food and junk food. You should also prepare your meals at home using fresh ingredients, instead of buying microwavable dishes.

Fast food, junk food, and processed foods are usually high in calories anyway. Nonetheless, even if you manage to avoid going beyond your calorie limit, the nutrients in these food products are still insufficient. Obviously, you will get sickly if your body lacks proper nutrients.

Do not forget to drink plenty of water daily. Water is essential in keeping your body hydrated. It does not have any calories, so you can have as much as you want. You may also drink herbal tea, black coffee, and even diet soda. Avoid beverages that are high in calories, such as milk.

Health should be your number one priority. When you aim to lose weight, you should only do so for the sake of your health. It is not wise to go on a diet and become underweight just because you want to look like a model. Dieting should be done to achieve and maintain your ideal weight and not for aesthetics.

Moreover, see to it that you get sufficient rest and sleep. Quit smoking, drinking liquor, doing drugs, or any other bad habits that you may have. Keep in mind that proper diet goes hand in hand with a healthy lifestyle. If you want to see good results, you should get your act right.

Benefits of the 5-2 Diet

For two days a week, you will only be consuming twenty-five percent of your normal calorie consumption. So in just a few weeks, you will already see noticeable results. The great thing about this diet is that you do not have to go on a diet every single day of the week.

With this diet, your body will not store more fat than it needs to. Hence, you will be able to prevent obesity. Keep in mind that being overweight or obese is not healthy, and can lead to a variety of life-threatening medical conditions.

The 5-2 diet also has other long-term benefits. For instance, it reduces levels of insulin-like growth factor 1 or IGF-1, which is the growth hormone responsible for making your body age. If you have healthy hormones, your body will be able to function at its best.

Likewise, you will be able to stay fresh, young-looking, and beautiful. You will be able to prevent developing cancer. The 5-2 diet can activate your DNA repair genes, as well as reduce your risks of high blood pressure and type 2 diabetes.

With this diet, you will also be able to reduce your levels of bad cholesterol and glucose. You will be able to improve your cognitive functions and avoid having Alzheimer's disease and dementia. You will also let your digestive system rest for a while.

Can Everyone Follow the 5-2 Diet?

The 5-2 diet is a generally safe diet. However, it may not be suitable for pregnant or lactating women and people with certain medical conditions. Diabetics, for instance, may experience unfavorable side effects if they follow this diet.

This is why it is crucial for you to consult your doctor before trying the 5-2 diet or any other diet program for that matter. See to it that you undergo the necessary tests, including blood test, in order to verify if you are indeed suitable for this diet.

If you go through the 5-2 diet and experience unpleasant side effects afterwards, seek medical attention immediately. Your doctor may advise you to discontinue this diet if you experience dizziness, irritability, headaches, lack of energy, and sleeping difficulty.

Breakfast Recipes

Breakfast is the most important meal of the day, which is why you should never skip it. If you do not have breakfast, you will not have enough energy to do your tasks or even think straight. When you are on the 5-2 diet, it is very important to choose what you eat wisely. For breakfast, you can have foods that contain one hundred calories or less. Here are some great examples:

A hardboiled or soft-boiled egg

One large egg typically contains a hundred calories. It is packed with protein, and it can keep you satiated until lunch time. It is also very easy to prepare. Just get an egg and boil it in a pot of water. If you want it to be tastier, you can eat it with some salt.

Scrambled egg with mushrooms

This meal contains about ninety-one calories. A medium egg typically contains seventy-eight calories while a hundred grams of chopped fresh mushrooms may contain thirteen calories. This breakfast is easy to prepare. Simply scramble the egg on a pan and add in the mushrooms. Do not use butter or milk. If you do not want the egg to stick to the pan, use a non-stick variety.

Spinach omelette

Omelette is another excellent meal you can prepare using an egg. This spinach omelette contains about ninety-four calories. A medium egg has seventy-eight calories and a sixty-gram spinach has sixteen calories. Egg is full of proteins while spinach is rich in iron. To prepare this meal, simply crack and whisk an egg and fry it on a pan, preferably the non-stick kind. When the bottom part of the omelette is already cooked, put the spinach in. Add some pepper, salt, and herbs to make the omelette tastier.

Ham omelette

If you are a meat lover, you can replace the spinach (from the spinach omelette recipe above) with ham. This ham omelette contains about ninety-seven calories. A medium egg contains seventy-eight calories while a slice of ham contains around nineteen calories. This delicious breakfast can be prepared in just five minutes. Simply cut the ham into tiny pieces and set aside. Crack and whisk an egg, and fry it. When the omelette is almost done, add the tiny pieces of ham to the pan. Take note that the smaller the pieces of ham are, the more flavorful your omelette can become. This breakfast is packed with protein, and can keep you full until lunch.

Beans on toast

If you want to eat toasted bread in the morning, you can prepare this simple breakfast. A slice of whole wheat bread only contains fifty-five calories and fifty grams of baked beans forty-two calories, summing up to ninety-seven calories. Just toast the bread, heat the beans, and you are all set.

Bread and honey

A slice of whole meal bread containing fifty-five calories plus two teaspoons of honey containing forty calories will give you ninety-five calories for breakfast. Bread and honey is perfect if you like toasted bread and are craving for something sweet. This light and tasty breakfast will satisfy your sweet tooth and give you the energy you need to start the day.

Banana and honey

If you love honey so much, you can also have it with banana. A small banana typically contains eighty-nine calories while half a teaspoon of honey contains ten calories. This very simple breakfast can give you ninety-nine calories. Just slice the banana into small chunks and drizzle it with honey. You can also mash up the banana and top it with honey.

Watermelon

Having fruits for breakfast is also ideal. A three hundred-gram slice of watermelon for instance, is light and naturally sweet. It contains ninety-six calories, and is much better than a cereal bar.

Blueberries, kiwi, and Greek yogurt

Blueberries and kiwi are fruits you should try too. You can mix them with Greek yogurt. Combine the ingredients in a bowl or put them in a food processor for a good yogurt smoothie. Fifty grams of blueberries contain twenty-nine calories while one chopped kiwi contains forty-two calories. Three tablespoons of fat-free Greek yogurt contains twenty-four calories. All in all, this breakfast contains ninety-five calories.

Apricot, mixed berries, and Greek Yogurt

Greek yogurt also goes well with apricots and berries, such as raspberries, strawberries, and blackberries. One apricot contains seventeen calories. Fifty grams of raspberries contain nineteen calories while fifty grams of strawberries contain sixteen calories. Fifty grams of blackberries contain twenty calories and three tablespoons of fat-free Greek yogurt contain twenty-four calories. This delicious blend of yogurt and fruits contain a total of ninety-six calories.

Sultanas, almonds, and Greek yogurt

Other ingredients you can mix with Greek yogurt are sultanas and almonds. A tablespoon of sultanas contains forty-two calories; four pieces of almonds contain twenty-eight calories; and three tablespoons of fat-free Greek yogurt contain twenty-four calories. This breakfast contains a total of ninety-four calories. To prepare this breakfast, start by crushing the almonds. Almonds are rich in healthy fats, which keep the body energetic and feeling full longer. Then, mix the crush almonds, the sultanas, and the Greek yogurt together. Enjoy.

Porridge

A bowl of porridge is an excellent way to begin your day. It contains oats that can keep you full until lunch time. Twenty-five grams of porridge oats contain eighty-nine calories and half a teaspoon of honey contains ten calories. This gives you ninety-nine calories for breakfast. In order for you to avoid going beyond your calorie limit, you should mix the oats with water instead of milk. Water does not contain any calories. You can also add a pinch of cinnamon to sweeten your porridge. Do not worry because the amount of calories contained in a pinch of cinnamon is negligible.

Lunch Recipes

Lunch is another important meal of the day. Therefore, it has to be packed with vital nutrients, so you can have enough energy to complete your tasks. It should also be satisfying enough to get you through until your next meal. Meat dishes are great, but soups and salads are also ideal for lunch. Since you are on the 5-2 diet, you should keep your calorie limit to two hundred calories. Here are excellent 5-2 diet lunch recipes you can try:

Chicken pitas (one hundred and sixty-two calories per serving)

✓ *Preparation time: twenty-five minutes*

✓ *Cooking time: ten minutes*

✓ *Total time: thirty-five minutes*

Ingredients:

1. Two tablespoons of low-fat yogurt

2. Two teaspoons of tomato puree

3. Two teaspoons of curry paste

4. One teaspoon of cooking oil

5. One hundred and fifty grams of skinless chicken breast or thigh (uncooked and cut into strips)

6. Two pita breads

7. Cherry tomatoes

8. Lettuce

Instructions:

Combine the curry paste, yogurt, and tomato puree together before adding in the chicken. When the chicken is coated, cover it and put it inside the refrigerator for fifteen minutes. While cooling the chicken, heat a non-stick pan and add oil. Place the chicken into the pan and fry over medium heat for five to eight minutes. Finally, shred the lettuce and add it into the pitta breads with the chicken. Serve it with tomatoes and other vegetables and fruits.

Pitta pizza made with smoked salmon (one hundred and ninety-four calories)

✓ *Preparation time: five minutes*

✓ *Cooking time: ten minutes*

✓ *Total time: fifteen minutes*

Ingredients:

1. One pitta bread
2. One tablespoon of low-fat cream cheese
3. One teaspoon of drained capers
4. One-fourth diced red onion
5. Lemon wedge
6. Lettuce
7. Dill

Instructions:

Preheat your oven to a hundred and eighty degrees Celsius. At the same time, spread some cream cheese into the pitta bread and add in pieces of smoked salmon. Sprinkle some red onions and capers on top. Put this in the oven and bake for ten minutes. When you see that the pitta bread is already crispy and golden, take it out of the oven. Serve it with fresh dill, lettuce, and a lemon wedge.

Crushed potatoes with shoots (one hundred and seventy calories)

✓ *Preparation time: fifteen minutes*

✓ *Cooking time: twenty-two minutes*

✓ *Total time: thirty-seven minutes*

Ingredients:

1. Five hundred grams of potatoes
2. One hundred grams of asparagus tips
3. One hundred grams of cooked petit pois
4. Eight hardboiled quail eggs
5. Two to four chopped spring onions
6. One lemon
7. Three tablespoons of olive oil
8. Pea shoots
9. Cress and mustard
10. Salt and pepper

Instructions:

Boil the potatoes in a pan of water with salt for fifteen to twenty minutes. When the potatoes are tender, add in the asparagus. Simmer for two more minutes before taking out the spears and refreshing them in cold water. Get the potatoes, cut them in halves, and use a fork to squash them. Get a jar and combine the lemon juice and oil to make the dressing. Then, pour it on the potatoes as you also add in the spring onions. On a plate, place the asparagus and potatoes. Add in the peas, eggs, and shoots. Place the cress and mustard on the edges of your plate. Add more of the dressing, and serve.

Orange, steak, and chicory (one hundred and seventy-nine calories)

✓ *Preparation time: ten minutes*

✓ *Cooking time: twelve minutes*

✓ *Total time: twenty-two minutes*

Ingredients:

11. Two pieces of one hundred and fifty-gram sirloin steaks

12. Two oranges

13. Six teaspoons of olive oil

14. Two teaspoons of vinegar

15. One teaspoon of mustard

16. Two heads of sliced white chicory

17. One head of radicchio or red chicory

18. One red onion

19. Wild rocket

20. Salt and pepper

Instructions:

Heat a pan over medium heat. At the same time, rub one teaspoon of olive oil on the steaks. Fry each side for about two minutes. Wrap them in foil. You have to slice these steaks later on. Boil orange juice in the pan until they become syrupy. Remove the heat and add in the mustard, vinegar, seasoning, and oil. Add the white chicory, red onion, and more oil. Cook them for several minutes until they become tender and brown in color. Combine all ingredients with the dressing and orange. Serve with the rocket and red chicory.

Red pepper soup (one hundred and twenty calories)

✓ *Preparation time: fifteen minutes*

✓ *Cooking time: thirty minutes*

✓ *Total time: forty-five minutes*

Ingredients:

1. Four large de-seeded and halved red peppers
2. Olive oil
3. Two diced onions
4. Four cloves of garlic
5. One finely diced red chili
6. Four hundred grams of canned tomatoes
7. One and a half liters of vegetable stock
8. One tablespoon of fennel seeds
9. Tabasco sauce
10. Thyme or basil leaves
11. Salt and pepper

Instructions:

Preheat your grill before grilling the red peppers. When you notice that they have already charred and blistered, get them out of the grill and place them inside a plastic bag to cool. Heat your saucepan and add in the oil. Cook the fennel seeds and onions together over medium heat for around five minutes. Peel off the skin of the peppers and chop their flesh. Add this to the other ingredients in your saucepan. Add all the other ingredients, except for the thyme or basil leaves. You will use these leaves for garnish later on. Boil the ingredients in the saucepan and simmer for fifteen to twenty minutes. Then, put them in your food processor or blender to liquidize them and make a soup. Place the soup back in the saucepan and adjust the seasoning. Finally, garnish it with thyme or basil leaves and serve with bread.

Roasted tomato and garlic soup (seventy calories)

- ✓ *Preparation time: five minutes*
- ✓ *Cooking time: fifty minutes*
- ✓ *Total time: fifty-five minutes*

Ingredients:

1. Low-fat oil
2. Five hundred grams of quartered tomatoes
3. Six hundred milliliters of vegetable stock
4. Two red onions cut into wedges
5. One bulb of garlic
6. One quartered and de-seeded red pepper
7. One tablespoon of Balsamic vinegar
8. One tablespoon of Worcestershire sauce
9. Basil leaves
10. Salt and pepper

Instructions:

Preheat your oven to two hundred and twenty degrees Celsius. Place the garlic, onions, red pepper, and tomatoes into a roasting tin and season with pepper and salt. Spray some low-fat oil and roast it for forty-five minutes or until the vegetables become soft and start to burn at the edges. Take the vegetables out of your oven and let them cool for several minutes. Then, place them in a food processor and make a purée. Do not forget to add the Balsamic vinegar, Worcestershire sauce, and vegetable stock. When the purée is done, transfer it into a medium-sized saucepan. Heat it for three to five minutes and serve with basil leaves. You can also serve it cold if you want.

Spring vegetable soup (one hundred and sixty-three calories)

✓ *Preparation time: fifteen minutes*

✓ *Cooking time: twenty minutes*

✓ *Total time: thirty-five minutes*

Ingredients:

1. One liter of chicken or vegetable stock
2. Two hundred grams of quartered baby potatoes
3. One hundred grams of halved baby carrots
4. One hundred grams of frozen or fresh peas
5. Twelve mint leaves
6. Three to four spring greens
7. Four chopped baby leeks
8. Two cloves of garlic
9. One chopped small onion
10. One sliced stick of celery

Instructions:

Boil the stock in a pan, and add the carrots, leeks, onion, garlic, and celery. Add the potatoes and simmer for twelve to fifteen minutes or until the potatoes are tender. Then, add the peas and the spring greens. The spring greens should be just under the stock. Simmer for five more minutes and serve. Sprinkle the chopped mint leaves as garnish.

Chicken miso soup (one hundred and thirty-two calories)

✓ *Preparation time: fifteen minutes*

✓ *Cooking time: ten minutes*

✓ *Total time: twenty-five minutes*

Ingredients:

1. Eight sliced shiitake mushrooms

2. Two sachets of Japanese miso paste, fifteen grams each

3. One sliced chicken breast

4. One crushed clove of garlic

5. One-half teaspoon of grated ginger

6. One-fourth of shredded cabbage

7. Soy sauce

Instructions:

Boil six hundred milliliters of water and transfer it into a medium-sized pan. Add in the sachets of miso paste and whisk. Then, add in the other ingredients except for cabbage. Simmer for about ten minutes. Finally, add in the cabbage and cook for three more minutes. Serve and enjoy.

Bean salad with tangy mustard dressing (one hundred and eighty calories)

✓ *Preparation time: twenty-five minutes*

✓ *Cooking time: five minutes*

✓ *Total time: thirty minutes*

Ingredients:

1. Four hundred grams of canned borlotti beans
2. Four hundred grams of canned cannellini beans
3. Ninety grams of halved green beans
4. Six cherry tomatoes
5. Two sticks of celery
6. One chopped red onion
7. Dressing ingredients:
8. Four tablespoons of olive oil
9. Two tablespoons of mustard
10. One tablespoon of honey
11. Lemon juice
12. Salt and pepper

Instructions:

Mix the green beans with two tablespoons of water in a microwavable container. Cover it and heat it inside the microwave oven for two minutes. Take the container out, rinse the green beans in cold water, and transfer them into a bowl. Rinse the red onion to get rid of its strong flavor. Add it to the bowl with the green beans. Add in the tomatoes, celery, and canned beans. For the dressing, mix together honey, lemon juice, olive oil, and mustard in a small container. Add some seasoning and shake. When the dressing is ready, drizzle it over the salad. Serve and enjoy.

Prawn and pickled cucumber salad (one hundred calories)

✓ *Preparation time: twenty-five minutes*

✓ *Cooking time: five minutes*

✓ *Total time: thirty minutes*

Ingredients:

1. Two hundred and eighty grams of tiger prawns
2. One cucumber
3. Three teaspoons of sesame oil
4. Two teaspoons of salt
5. Baby spinach
6. Dressing Ingredients:
7. One clove of garlic
8. One-half red chili
9. Four tablespoons of lime juice
10. Two tablespoons of chopped coriander leaves
11. One tablespoon of chopped mint leaves
12. One tablespoon of fish sauce
13. One teaspoon of brown sugar

Instructions:

Cut the cucumber into tiny diagonal pieces and put inside a colander. Sprinkle some salt and mix it in. Leave it for about an hour. Prepare the dressing by whisking all ingredients in a bowl. Wash the cucumber and dry it using a clean towel, and then add it to the dressing. Gently stir the cucumber with the dressing. Taste it and add more seasoning if you want. Put the spinach in a bowl and add in the pickled cucumber. Preheat a pan and add a teaspoon of sesame oil. Cook the prawns for several minutes until they become pinkish in color. When they are done, spoon them over your salad. Sprinkle more sesame oil and add in any remaining dressing. Garnish your salad with the chopped coriander leaves and serve.

Dinner Recipes

A lot of dieters believe that skipping dinner can make them lose weight faster. However, this is not a very good idea. Skipping dinner can be bad for your health. If you want to lose weight and still be healthy, you should count your calories. Dinner is something that you should look forward to at the end of the day. Reward yourself and have a great meal after a hard day's work. The 5-2 diet suggests that you consume up to two hundred or three hundred calories for dinner. Here are some amazing recipes you can try:

Chinese vegetable chowmein (one hundred and seventy calories)

✓ *Preparation time: fifteen minutes*

✓ *Cooking time: five minutes*

✓ *Total time: twenty minutes*

Ingredients:

1. Three hundred grams of egg noodles

2. One hundred and twenty-five grams of oyster mushrooms

3. One hundred and twenty-five grams of broccoli

4. Two tablespoons of vegetable oil

5. One or two tablespoons of oyster sauce

6. One tablespoon of soy sauce

7. One tablespoon of rice vinegar

8. One sliced red pepper

9. One sliced carrot

One lime

Instructions:

Preheat a large pan and add the vegetable oil. Cook all the vegetables for two to three minutes, and then add the oyster sauce, soy sauce, and rice vinegar. Add the egg noodles and cook some more. Transfer to a plate and squeeze the lime juice on top. Serve and enjoy.

Roasted ratatouille (one hundred and fifty calories)

✓ *Preparation time: twenty minutes*

✓ *Cooking time: one hour*

✓ *Total time: one hour and twenty minutes*

Ingredients:

1. Four hundred grams of chopped tomatoes

2. Four large, halved round or plum tomatoes

3. Two cut, halved, and deseeded bell peppers

4. Two cloves of garlic

5. Two halved courgettes

6. Two red onions

7. One thickly sliced aubergine

8. Five tablespoons of olive oil

9. One tablespoon of dried oregano

10. Salt and pepper

Instructions:

Preheat your oven to one hundred and ninety degrees Celsius. Place all the vegetables in a roasting tin or tray. Arrange them in just one layer. Sprinkle some seasoning, oregano, and olive oil. Use your hand to mix all the ingredients. Roast for forty-five to fifty minutes until the vegetables become soft and brownish in color. Stir a few times and wait until the vegetables are almost done. In a separate pan, cook the garlic until they turn brown. Add in the tomatoes and cook for ten minutes. Add the vegetables into the pan with the tomatoes.

Fish burger (one hundred and forty-one calories)

✓ *Preparation time: ten minutes*

✓ *Cooking time: six minutes*

✓ *Total time: sixteen minutes*

Ingredients:

1. Four hundred grams of fish fillet

2. Five tablespoons of chopped parsley

3. One tablespoon of capers

4. One tablespoon of olive oil

5. Lemon zest

6. Flour

7. Salt and pepper

Instructions:

Cut the fish fillet into tiny pieces or place it inside a food processor. Add in the capers, parsley, seasoning, and lemon zest. Use your hand to mix all the ingredients thoroughly and shape them into circles. Put the burgers inside the refrigerator and chill them until firm. Preheat a pan and add the oil. Sprinkle some flour on the burgers before frying them over low or medium heat. Cook each side for three minutes or until brown. Serve with bread or salad.

Udon noodles and Japanese broth (two hundred and fifty calories)

✓ *Preparation time: five minutes*

✓ *Cooking time: fifteen minutes*

✓ *Total time: twenty minutes*

Ingredients:

1. Two hundred and fifty grams of mixed mushrooms (shiitake, button, and oyster)

2. One hundred and seventy grams of rice or udon noodles

3. One hundred and fifty grams of fillet steak

4. One hundred grams of mange tout

5. One and a half liters of beef or vegetable stock

6. One sachet of miso paste

7. Two spring onions

8. One clove of garlic

9. One red chili

10. One to two tablespoons of soy sauce or fish sauce

11. Ginger root slices

12. Lime wedges

Instructions:

Boil some water and salt in a pan, and add in the noodles. After six to eight minutes, drain the noodles and rinse them in cold water. Set aside for a while. Get another pan and heat the ginger and stock. Add in soy sauce or fish sauce and miso paste, and boil the ingredients. Add in the mushrooms, chili, and garlic. Simmer for three minutes. Add in the meat and mange tout. Simmer for two minutes and add seasoning for added flavor. Place the noodles in a bowl and pour over the broth. Sprinkle some spring onions or serve immediately with the lime wedges.

Moroccan tomatoes (two hundred and twenty-one calories)

✓ *Preparation time: five minutes*

✓ *Cooking time: ten minutes*

✓ *Total time: fifteen minutes*

Ingredients:

1. One hundred grams of asparagus

2. Two medium eggs

3. One large tomato

4. One clove of garlic

5. Two tablespoons of olive oil

6. Cumin or paprika

7. Salt and pepper

Instructions:

Preheat a pan and add the olive oil. Cook the asparagus for two minutes and add in the garlic. Cook them for one minute, and add in slices of tomato. Cook for two more minutes. Crack the eggs open over the pan. Place a lid on top and wait until the eggs have set according to your preference. Sprinkle some salt and pepper to taste. Serve with bread and enjoy.

Chorizo and squash stew (two hundred and sixty-four calories)

✓ *Preparation time: ten minutes*

✓ *Cooking time: twenty-five minutes*

✓ *Total time: thirty-five minutes*

Ingredients:

1. One hundred and forty grams of sliced chorizo

2. Six hundred and eighty grams of pasta

3. One chopped onion

4. One butternut squash cut into tiny chunks

5. Parsley

Instructions:

Preheat a pan, add in the chorizo slices, and cook over high heat for two minutes. When oil is released from the chorizo, set the slices aside and add in the onion. Fry for five minutes. Add in the squash, chorizo, and pasta. Boil for fifteen to twenty minutes or until the squash becomes soft but still intact. Add some seasoning and garnish with parsley. Serve and enjoy.

Snack and Dessert Ideas

Believe it or not, eating snacks and desserts will not be a hindrance to your weight loss goals. In fact, snacking can help you avoid hunger pangs throughout the day. Indulging in delicious desserts is also allowed. Just make sure that you do not exceed your daily calorie limit. Here are awesome 5-2 snack and dessert suggestions for you:

Carrot sticks and humus

You can eat one-fourth tub of low-fat humus and four carrot sticks for an afternoon snack. This gives you one hundred calories.

Toasted crumpets

Baked goods are usually not ideal if you are on a diet. However, a toasted crumpet with low-fat cheese can make an excellent snack with only one hundred calories. Just make sure that you avoid using butter.

A pear

Pears are refreshing and rich in vitamins. A medium pear can give you one hundred calories.

Sweet Corn on the cob

A corn on the cob is highly recommended in the summer. Sprinkle over some salt for added taste. This snack also gives you one hundred calories.

Jellybeans

If you are craving for sweets, you can reach for twenty-five pieces of jellybeans that contain one hundred calories in total.

Almonds

Almonds are excellent for snacking. They are nutritious and delicious. You can have fourteen pieces for ninety-eight calories.

Bananas

Frozen or fresh, bananas are great for snacking or dessert. One banana gives you ninety-five calories.

Mangoes

Four mango slices give you just ninety calories. So if you want to have a sweet treat after dinner, you can have a mango.

Marshmallows

Four pieces of marshmallows can also give you ninety calories. You can eat them straight from the bag or toast them. You can also add them in your cup of hot cocoa.

Blueberries

These berries are tasty and healthy. They are great for both snacks and dessert. A cup of these gives you eighty-three calories.

Chocolate-coated raisins

If you think that you can no longer have chocolate for dessert, think again. Raisins coated in chocolate are really great-tasting and have only eighty calories.

Peaches

Peaches are rich in vitamins, and helpful in reducing levels of cholesterol and regenerating skin tissues. They are very delicious, as well. A couple of medium peaches can give you seventy-six calories.

Olives

If you are in search of a low-calorie wine partner, you can nibble twenty pieces of olives. Olives are way better and more nutritious than crisps. Twenty pieces of olives contain just sixty-eight calories.

Highlights Mousse by Cadbury

Chocolate mousse is a common dessert. It is sweet and heavenly. If you are craving for one, you can have Highlights Mousse for only sixty calories. This sweet dessert will not leave you feeling guilty.

Strawberries

Sixteen pieces of strawberries can give you fifty-eight calories. So the next time you feel like snacking, grab some strawberries. They are especially ideal during summer.

Blackberries

These berries can easily be found at your local supermarket. They are sweet and rich in antioxidants. Twenty pieces of blackberries can give you forty-eight calories.

Conclusion

Thank you again for downloading this book!

I hope this book was able to help you to understand how the 5-2 diet works as well as learn new recipes.

The next step is to go to the supermarket and start trying out these amazing recipes.

Finally, if you enjoyed this book, please take the time to share your thoughts and post a review on Amazon. It'd be greatly appreciated!

Thank you and good luck!

Made in the USA
Monee, IL
18 April 2025

16042035R00026